Distribution, publication, and copying in any form are prohibited and subject to damages.

## TEN HYPNOSES

Copying, publishing, and sharing with third parties are only permitted with the written consent of the author. Please observe the notes on copyright and usage.

Distribution, publication, and copying in any form are prohibited and subject to damages.

Copying, publishing, and sharing with third parties are only permitted with the written consent of the author. Please observe the notes on copyright and usage.

Distribution, publication, and copying in any form are prohibited and subject to damages.

Ingo Michael Simon

# TEN HYPNOSES

18

ANTI-VIOLENCE TRAINING, OFFENDER SUPPORT

Copying, publishing, and sharing with third parties are only permitted with the written consent of the author. Please observe the notes on copyright and usage.

Distribution, publication, and copying in any form are prohibited and subject to damages.

© 2024 Ingo Michael Simon
All rights reserved.
Independently published
www.ingosimon.com

Important Notes for Urgent Attention:
The contents of this book are based on the practical experiences of the author with hypnosis applications and psychotherapy in a trance state. Although the author has strived for the utmost care, errors or misunderstandings in the presentation cannot be completely excluded. Therapeutic work with people and the application of hypnosis are solely the responsibility of the hypnotist. It cannot be ruled out that parts of this book may be misunderstood or that the application of a presented procedure may cause an undesirable reaction in the client. The author also assumes no co-responsibility if work with a client is carried out with reference to the statements in this book.

The Author:
Ingo Michael Simon studied psychology and education and is a hypnotherapist with practices in southwestern Germany and Switzerland. With the help of hypnosis-supported psychotherapy, he primarily treats people with persistent psychological conditions. His practice focuses on anxiety disorders, pathological compulsions, and psychosomatic illnesses. His therapeutic offerings mainly include classical and modern hypnosis applications and the dreamland therapy he developed himself.

Copying, publishing, and sharing with third parties are only permitted with the written consent of the author. Please observe the notes on copyright and usage.

Distribution, publication, and copying in any form are prohibited and subject to damages.

## Notes on Copyright and Usage

Copying, publishing, and sharing with third parties is prohibited and only permitted with the written consent of the author. Please observe the following copyright and usage guidelines.

This work has been carefully crafted and created to the best of the author's knowledge and personal experience. It comprises text templates and application guidelines for professional hypnosis sessions. The author is a licensed psychotherapist with extensive experience in psychotherapy, coaching, and personal training using hypnotic techniques and methods. Nevertheless, the author and the publisher assume no liability for the accuracy of information, instructions, and advice, nor for any typographical errors. The author and publisher accept no responsibility or liability for the application of these texts and recommendations with clients or patients, nor for any potential consequences or unexpected reactions. It is expressly noted that the application of therapeutic and advisory techniques and formulations lies solely and entirely within the responsibility of the practitioner. This also applies to adherence to the boundaries of legally regulated medical and therapeutic practices. The fact that a book containing action proposals is freely available for sale does not imply that its application with clients or patients is permitted for everyone.

Copying, publishing, and sharing with third parties are only permitted with the written consent of the author. Please observe the notes on copyright and usage.

Distribution, publication, and copying in any form are prohibited and subject to damages.

Copying, publishing, and sharing with third parties are only permitted with the written consent of the author. Please observe the notes on copyright and usage.

Distribution, publication, and copying in any form are prohibited and subject to damages.

## Table of Contents

Introduction ................................................................................................. 9

#1 ............................................................................................................. 11

#2 ............................................................................................................. 16

#3 ............................................................................................................. 23

#4 ............................................................................................................. 29

#5 ............................................................................................................. 33

#6 ............................................................................................................. 40

#7 ............................................................................................................. 46

#8 ............................................................................................................. 51

#9 ............................................................................................................. 57

#10 ........................................................................................................... 64

Overview of All Titles in the Series "Ten Hypnoses" ........................................ 70

Copying, publishing, and sharing with third parties are only permitted with the written consent of the author. Please observe the notes on copyright and usage.

Distribution, publication, and copying in any form are prohibited and subject to damages.

Copying, publishing, and sharing with third parties are only permitted with the written consent of the author. Please observe the notes on copyright and usage.

## Introduction

The series "Ten Hypnoses" is very well known in Germany, Austria, and Switzerland as a collection of texts for therapeutic work and is used by numerous psychotherapeutic practices, doctors, therapists, coaches, and other helping professionals. I am pleased to now be able to offer these texts in other countries as well.

Most therapists have their own methods for inducing and deepening trance as well as for exiting trance. Therefore, I have focused on the main part of the hypnosis. The texts in this book can be integrated as the main part into any hypnosis process.

The texts in this collection use various hypnosis techniques. I will not explain these in detail, as I assume that users have the appropriate training. It is also not necessary to understand the exact structure or functioning of the different parts. The texts can simply be read aloud, and they will have their effect.

Decide for yourself which text best suits your client or patient at any given time. You can also combine passages from different texts. It is not about using all ten hypnoses in sequence. It is a selection of possibilities.

I want to emphasize that books cannot replace therapy. Psychotherapy or other therapeutic treatments involve much more. A careful diagnosis is the necessary basis for deciding on the use of methods, including whether hypnosis or one of my texts should be used. Even in this case, preparatory discussions, follow-up discussions during the session, and of course, a therapeutic concept for the sequence of sessions and the content approaches are essential parts of therapy. This cannot and should not be achieved with a collection of texts.

In any case, I wish you much success in your work and I am pleased if my text templates can contribute in a small way.

*Ingo Michael Simon*

# #1

### Contact and Relief

... ... You are a perpetrator ... ... You have committed violence ... ... more extreme and frequent than could be justified ... ... You know this yourself because you have realized that you must stop ... ... you know and always knew that it was wrong ... ... Surely, for a while, you found some official justification for yourself and presented it to others ... ... you blamed the victims of your violence for your actions ... ... you claimed they provoked you and thus started the conflict ... ... and if they hadn't done that, it wouldn't have happened ... ... The other person started it ... ... You know this ... ... You yourself know best that these could never really justify violence ... ... The good thing is, you have come to realize that it was wrong ... ... You have been condemned by many, maybe even by a court ... ... but not only there ... ... and now you condemn the violence yourself ... ... You hold yourself accountable and responsible to change ... ... Three steps are necessary for this ... ... first, you must take responsibility for your actions, without excuses ... ... You have already done this, so you have taken the first step and can move forward seriously ... ... the second step is to decide against violence ... ... You have also taken this step, deciding against violence ... ... Your challenge now is to stand by this decision and act accordingly ... ... and that is why you are here ... ... to help yourself ... ... to never be a perpetrator again ... ... The third step is to deal with your own past, because you were once a victim of violence yourself ... ... Violence made you a perpetrator ... ... or better yet ... ... violence invited you to repeat what happened to you, but it's up to you to break this cycle ... ...

Self-Forgiveness and Comfort

... ... So you have taken responsibility for yourself ... ... and you know that violence is wrong, but it's also time for you to forgive yourself ... ... This is not easy, and maybe you think it is inappropriate or others think so ... ... But forgiveness does not mean that you condone what you have done ... ... You are determined to take responsibility for your actions and change your life ... ... If you can eventually forgive yourself, then the violence can completely stop ... ... because only as a free person can you freely decide against violence ... ... and you do not want to speak out against violence out of guilt but out of conviction ... ... So try to forgive yourself ... ... Try to understand that in the past you simply could not break away from the model of violence ... ... Try at least to forgive the child in you ... ... the child you once were and who experienced violence and felt guilty ... ... But as a child, you were not guilty or responsible ... ... Comfort the beaten child within you ... ... [approximately 20 seconds of silence] ... ...

Resolution and Self-Agreement

+++ Variant 1: General Use of Violence +++

... ... You can make an agreement with yourself ... ... a pact of peace ... ... You make peace with the past by accepting that you cannot change your own history ... ... you cannot undo your actions either ... ... You make peace with yourself and accept the fear and sadness of your childhood memories and at the same time accept that you are now an adult ... ... Despite all the understandable suffering of your childhood, your violence did nothing for the child within you ... ... Violence makes everything worse ... ... So make peace with the child within you ... ... Comfort it and be there for it ... ... And make peace with your victims ... ... They were just as innocent as the child back then ... ... Make peace and then resolve not to make anyone a victim anymore ... ... no one should pay for your childhood ... ... not even you ... ...

+++ End of Variant 1 +++

+++ Variant 2: Convicted Violent Offenders +++

... ... You can make an agreement with yourself ... ... a pact of loyalty ... ... You can be loyal to yourself ... ... to your feelings, the feelings of the child who once experienced violence ... ... As a child, you wished the violence would end ... ... maybe you prayed for it or sought help and did not get it ... ... because no one was there to recognize your distress or could recognize it ... ... or those who recognized your distress could or would not help you ... ... for whatever reason ... ... It was as it was ... ... But the child wished for a world without violence, longed for it ... ... Fulfill this child's dream within you ... ... and free your life from your violence ... ... Make a pact of loyalty with the child ... ...

+++ End of Variant 2 +++

Success and Reinforcement

… … Now stay a little longer in the tranquility of the trance … … You have already achieved a lot because you are on a new path … … on the way to yourself, to your deepest feelings, and they lead you far away from any violence … … And with this first step, which is much bigger than you think, it will be much easier for you now to really come to terms with your experiences and make a clean break with violence … … ending violence through responsibility … … ending violence through a clear decision against it … … ending violence through dealing with your own life story … … You can do it … … Yes, you can do it … …

# #2

## Goal Formulation and Will Strengthening

… … I am finally ready to take full responsibility for my actions … … that is why I can distance myself from violence … …

… … I am finally ready to take full responsibility for my actions … … that is why I face the past and change my behavior … …

… … I am finally ready to take full responsibility for my actions … … that is why I respect the right to the integrity of others … …

… … I am finally ready to take full responsibility for my actions … … that is why I fully engage in this hypnosis … …

## Thought Orientation

+++ Variant 1: General Use of Violence +++

... ... I know that I am responsible for everything I do ... ... and therefore I can recognize what I have caused with violence ... ...

... ... I know that I am responsible for everything I do ... ... and therefore I can now also consciously separate myself from violence ... ...

... ... I know that I am responsible for everything I do ... ... and therefore only I can make a clear decision against violence ... ...

... ... I know that I am responsible for everything I do ... ... and therefore it is now time to end the violence ... ...

... ... I end the violence ... ... yes, I end the violence ... ... Now ... ...

+++ End of Variant 1 +++

### +++ Variant 2: Convicted Violent Offenders +++

... ... I know that I was rightly convicted by a court ... ... and therefore I can recognize what I have caused with violence ... ...

... ... I know that I was rightly convicted by a court ... ... and therefore I can now also consciously separate myself from violence ... ...

... ... I know that I was rightly convicted by a court ... ... and therefore only I can make a clear decision against violence ... ...

... ... I know that I was rightly convicted by a court ... ... and therefore it is now time to end the violence and start a better life ... ...

... ... I end the violence ... ... yes, I end the violence ... ... Now ... ...

+++ End of Variant 2 +++

## Somatic Orientation

... ... My body is now in healing calm and relaxation ... ... therefore I also feel that the wounds of the past are healing more and more ... ...

... ... My body is now in healing calm and relaxation ... ... therefore I recognize in all calmness what I really need to change my life ... ...

... ... My body is now in healing calm and relaxation ... ... therefore I can now also feel that I need self-confidence to end the violence ...

... ... My body is now in healing calm and relaxation ... ... therefore I can especially recognize that calmness and composure are the right way for me ... ...

... ... I end the violence ... ... yes, I end the violence ... ... Now ... ...

## Emotional Orientation

... ... I am self-confident and strong, especially without violence ... ... and that is why I can also let go of the violence ... ...

… … I am self-confident and strong, especially without violence … … and that is why I really want to live without violence … …

… … I am self-confident and strong, especially without violence … … and that is why I now really stand up for a life completely without violence … …

… … I am self-confident and strong, especially without violence … … and that is why this is my life path … … taking responsibility and ending violence … …

… … I end the violence … … yes, I end the violence … … Now … …


Behavioral Orientation

… … I actively and confidently advocate for a peaceful and constructive coexistence … … because I am responsible for my actions, only I alone … …

… … I actively and confidently advocate for a peaceful and constructive coexistence … … because this is how I truly take responsibility in my life … …

… … I actively and confidently advocate for a peaceful and constructive coexistence … … because this is how I can and will prove that I can resolve conflicts constructively … …

… … I actively and confidently advocate for a peaceful and constructive coexistence … … because this is how I can also successfully process all aggressive impulses …

… … I end the violence … … yes, I end the violence … … Now … …


Reinforcement

… … I fully align myself with a non-violent life, and with each new day, it becomes easier for me to reject violence … … and by doing so, I show real strength and real responsibility …

… … I fully align myself with a non-violent life, and with each new day, it becomes easier for me to reject violence … … and that makes me much more self-confident and stronger than violence ever could … …

… … I fully align myself with a non-violent life, and with each new day, it becomes easier for me to reject violence …

... because I have made my decision ... ... I have chosen a constructive life ... ... without violence ... ... completely without violence ... ...

# #3

## Goal Formulation and Will Strengthening

... ... I find deep peace today in this trance and deep within myself ... ... because this is the quickest way for me to separate from violence and start a new life ...

... ... I am determined to let all suggestions take effect ... ... because this is the quickest way for me to separate from violence and start a new life ... ...

... ... I am ready to truly accept helpful words ... ... because this is the quickest way for me to separate from violence and start a new life ... ...

... ... I fully engage in this helpful hypnosis today ... ... because this is the quickest way for me to separate from violence and start a new life ... ...

## Thought Orientation

### +++ Variant 1: General Use of Violence +++

... ... I know that serenity begins in my own thoughts ... ... and with this thought, I can repeatedly let go of aggressive impulses ... ...

... ... I know that I can decide for myself what I do ... ... and with this thought, I can repeatedly let go of aggressive impulses ... ...

... ... I know that I can consciously decide against violence ... ... and with this thought, I can repeatedly let go of aggressive impulses ... ...

... ... I know that my violence has always hit innocent people ... ... and with this thought, I can repeatedly let go of aggressive impulses ... ...

... ... I now decide for a peaceful and responsible life ... ...

+++ End of Variant 1 +++

+++ Variant 2: Convicted Violent Offenders +++

... ... I know that violence is rightly a crime ... ... and with this thought, I can repeatedly let go of aggressive impulses and not be a perpetrator ... ...

... ... I know that I can decide for myself what I do ... ... and with this thought, I can repeatedly let go of aggressive impulses and not be a perpetrator ... ...

... ... I never want to inflict the injustice of violence on others again ... ... and with this thought, I can repeatedly let go of aggressive impulses and not be a perpetrator ...

... ... I want to respect others' right to integrity ... ... and with this thought, I can repeatedly let go of aggressive impulses and not be a perpetrator ... ...

... ... I now decide for a peaceful and responsible life ... ...

+++ End of Variant 2 +++

## Somatic Orientation

… … The external posture of the body reflects the inner attitude … … and therefore I can have a calm demeanor and presence … …

… … My body can immediately adopt a calm and peaceful posture … … and therefore I can have a calm demeanor and presence … …

… … My body is now adopting a very relaxed and peaceful posture … … and therefore I can have a calm demeanor and presence … …

… … My body maintains this calm posture even in my everyday life … … and therefore I can have a calm demeanor and presence … …

… … I now decide for a peaceful and responsible life … …

## Emotional Orientation

… … I can now feel my own feelings better … … and therefore I feel that aggressive impulses have only to do with myself … …

… … I also feel that I lacked self-confidence … … and therefore I feel that aggressive impulses have only to do with myself … …

… … I feel that I rejected and despised myself … … and therefore I feel that aggressive impulses have only to do with myself … …

… … I accept my feelings, especially my self-worth problems … … and therefore I feel that aggressive impulses have only to do with myself … …

… … I now decide for a peaceful and responsible life … …

Behavioral Orientation

… … I will now actively work on my self-esteem … … I say no to all forms of violence and clearly yes to peaceful, constructive conflict resolution … …

… … I will now actively work on my self-confidence … … I say no to all forms of violence and clearly yes to peaceful, constructive conflict resolution … …

… … I will now work on my self-control … … I say no to all forms of violence and clearly yes to peaceful, constructive conflict resolution … …

… … I take full responsibility for my violence … … I say no to all forms of violence and clearly yes to peaceful, constructive conflict resolution … …

… … I now decide for a peaceful and responsible life … …

Reinforcement

… … The words I have heard are having a deeper and deeper effect … … and therefore I overcome the violence and leave it behind once and for all … … I take full responsibility for everything I have done and for everything I will do from now on … …

… … As soon as I am fully awake again, I will recognize even more clearly that I finally want to be free and I realize that I am indeed ready to end the violence forever … … I say no to all forms of violence and clearly yes to peaceful, constructive conflict resolution … … This is my path … … Yes, this is my path … …

# #4

## Contact and Relief

... ... You have made an important decision ... ... You have decided against violence ... ... You yourself have decided that it should finally stop ... ... Now it is up to you to fully put this into practice ... ... This means you need to control aggressive impulses ... ... You need methods and techniques to avoid confrontations that used to lead to violence ... ... and you need methods to prevent stress and pressure from building up in you in the first place ... ... Your new methods must have nothing to do with violence or destruction ... ... You have surely learned some things on this path and you are surely ready to take advantage of training to get better and better at it ... ... Training is part of it ... ... You know this because you need and want to learn to deal with your personality differently ... ... You are on a good path to achieving this ... ... You are also using this hypnosis and others because you are ready to look deeply into your emotions and make peace within ... ... Certainly a big step, because the violence was also used to avoid exactly that ...

… So you have come a long way … … Now it is mainly about a clear decision against violence and at the same time living this new basic attitude in your daily life … …

Self-Forgiveness and Comfort

… … You have already dealt a lot with your victims … … with their feelings and their suffering … … with the consequences of your violence … … And you have also dealt with yourself … … in your thoughts … … in conversations with therapists … … in confrontation with trainers who help you control and let go of the violence … … and also in your feelings … … in the introspection you hold during hypnosis … … That was also a strenuous path … … and for the fact that you are not only willing to walk it but actively and consciously do so, you can now also thank yourself … … You can and should thank the part of you that has decided against violence … … Maybe it sometimes struggles with another, impulsive, and still violent part … … But there is exactly this part of you that is ready to end the violence forever … … and you can now express your thanks to it … … … [approximately 20 seconds of silence] … …

## Resolution and Self-Agreement

+++ Variant 1: General Use of Violence +++

... ... You are strong enough to confront yourself and your actions ... ... and to speak out against violence ... ... You have officially and surely also out of conviction decided against violence ... ... Today you express it as a self-agreement inwardly ... ... to remind yourself and to make it an indelible and honest pact ... ... a permanent pact with yourself against violence ... ... You now agree with yourself to renounce violence forever ... ... You commit yourself before yourself to never use violence again and never to hit or threaten a person again ... ... never to commit violence against a person again ... ...

+++ End of Variant 1 +++

+++ Variant 2: Convicted Violent Offenders +++

... ... You are strong enough to confront yourself, your actions, and the court judgment you received for them ... ... and to now speak out against violence ... ... You have officially and surely also out of conviction decided against violence ... ... Today you express it as a self-agreement inwardly ... ... to remind yourself and to make it an indelible and honest pact … … a permanent pact with yourself and with all your victims … … your anti-violence pact … … You now agree with yourself and with all your victims to renounce violence forever … … You commit yourself before yourself and in respect of the suffering of your victims to never use violence again and never to hit or threaten a person again … … never to commit violence against a person again … … never to become a perpetrator again … …

+++ End of Variant 2 +++


Success and Reinforcement

… … Now let your pact sink into the depths of your subconscious so that a deep and honest pact against violence is created within you … … so that it becomes your deep and honest basic attitude to never become a perpetrator again … … never to hit or attack a person again … … Focus now on the relaxation of your body … … and if you think you could relax even more, then let go even more and relax your body … … because in true relaxation your pact will become a deep basic attitude the fastest ... ... just like that ... ... That's right ... ... It works ... ...

# #5

## Goal Formulation and Will Strengthening

… … I leave the time of violent outbursts behind me now … … because I have dealt with it and am ready to consciously and actively take new paths … …

… … I leave the time of violent outbursts behind me now … … because I have looked at and continue to process the past events and now want to be free again … …

… … I leave the time of violent outbursts behind me now … … because I internally set myself up to look forward and change everything … …

… … I leave the time of violent outbursts behind me now … … because I gain new thoughts and insights with this trance and can now take this step … …

## Thought Orientation

+++ Variant 1: General Use of Violence +++

... ... I know that it now comes down to my clear decision, so I decide ... ... and commit to rejecting all forms of violence ... ...

... ... I know that it now comes down to my clear decision, so I decide ... ... and commit to training my non-violent conflict resolution skills ... ...

... ... I know that it now comes down to my clear decision, so I decide ... ... and commit to working through my own memories of violence ... ...

... ... I know that it now comes down to my clear decision, so I decide ... ... and commit to doing everything to avoid violence now and in the future ... ...

... ... I have decided ... ... Never again violence ... ... Never again violence ... ...

+++ End of Variant 1 +++

+++ Variant 2: Convicted Violent Offenders +++

... ... I know that it now comes down to a new path and my personal probation ... ... and my path leads away from crimes and violence ... ...

... ... I know that it now comes down to a new path and my personal probation ... ... and therefore I continue to actively work on my self-control ... ...

... ... I know that it now comes down to a new path and my personal probation ... ... and therefore I finally process my own experiences of violence ... ...

... ... I know that it now comes down to a new path and my personal probation ... ... and therefore I truly end the violence today ... ...

... ... I have decided ... ... Never again violence ... ... Never again violence ... ...

+++ End of Variant 2 +++

## Somatic Orientation

... ... I feel the calm and relaxation of my body at this moment ... ... and I want this calm to become deep inner peace ... ... Now ... ...

... ... I feel the calm and relaxation of my body at this moment ... ... and I want this calm to become my inner peace even in conflicts and disputes ...

... ... I feel the calm and relaxation of my body at this moment ... ... and I want to always feel enough calm to stay without violence ... ...

... ... I feel the calm and relaxation of my body at this moment ... ... and I want to meet my fellow human beings with exactly this calm and relaxation ... ...

... ... I have decided ... ... Never again violence ... ... Never again violence ... ...

## Emotional Orientation

... ... I clearly feel that the relaxation and peace of the trance are good for me ... ... and I also respect everyone's right to peace and relaxation ... ...

... ... I clearly feel that the relaxation and peace of the trance are good for me ... ... and I respect everyone's right to peace and integrity ... ...

... ... I clearly feel that the relaxation and peace of the trance are good for me ... ... and I respect everyone's right to a non-violent life ... ...

... ... I clearly feel that the relaxation and peace of the trance are good for me ... ... and I decide now for relaxation and against violence ... ...

... ... I have decided ... ... Never again violence ... ... Never again violence ... ...

### Behavioral Orientation

... ... I say no to violence with full conviction and as my personal statement ... ... because this frees me from the past and allows me to move forward freely ... ...

... ... I say no to violence with full conviction and as my personal statement ... ... because this allows me to overcome past events and come to peace ... ...

… … I say no to violence with full conviction and as my personal statement … … because this reminds me of my goal of non-violence … …

… … I say no to violence with full conviction and as my personal statement … … because this prepares me for new freedom and new opportunities … …

… … I have decided … … Never again violence … … Never again violence … …

Reinforcement

… … I am and remain on a non-violent path, now and every day without violence … … because my decision against acts of violence and for a peaceful life stands firm … …

… … I am and remain on a non-violent path, now and every day without violence … … and I remain on my path of peace … … I have changed my attitude and I have changed my life … … I continue my path without violence … … completely without violence and I respect and protect my fellow human beings from arising aggressive impulses by avoiding confrontations ... ... This is my path ... ... Yes, this is my path ... ...

# #6

Goal Formulation and Will Strengthening

... ... I find deep peace today in this trance and deep within myself ... ... because this is how I remain steadfast in my decision to never be a perpetrator again ... ...

... ... I am determined to hear and let all suggestions take effect ... ... because this is how I remain steadfast in my decision to never be a perpetrator again ... ...

... ... I am ready to take in helpful words deep into my inner self ... ... because this is how I remain steadfast in my decision to never be a perpetrator again ... ...

... ... Today, I embark on a new path with the help of this hypnosis ... ... because this is how I remain steadfast in my decision to never be a perpetrator again ... ...

## Thought Orientation

### +++ Variant 1: General Use of Violence +++

... ... I know that innocent people became victims of my violence ... ... and this thought strengthens my decision to never use violence again ... ...

... ... I know that I oppressed and humiliated people ... ... and this thought strengthens my decision to never use violence again ... ...

... ... I know that I caused severe pain to people ... ... and this thought strengthens my decision to never use violence again ... ...

... ... I know that I caused fear and terror in people ... ... and this thought strengthens my decision to never use violence again ... ...

... ... I now decide to never use violence again ... ...

+++ End of Variant 1 +++

+++ Variant 2: Convicted Violent Offenders +++

… … I know that innocent people became victims of my violence … … and therefore I regret my actions and do everything to never be a perpetrator again … …

… … I know that I oppressed and humiliated people … … and therefore I regret my actions and do everything to never be a perpetrator again … …

… … I know that I caused severe pain to people … … and therefore I regret my actions and do everything to never be a perpetrator again … …

… … I know that I caused fear and terror in people … … and therefore I regret my actions and do everything to never be a perpetrator again … …

… … I now decide to never use violence again … …

+++ End of Variant 2 +++

## Somatic Orientation

...... My body is now completely relaxed, and this relaxation spreads further ...... and my body can also store peace and relaxation in every cell ......

...... Through simple inhalation and exhalation, my body was able to relax so deeply ...... and my body can also store peace and relaxation in every cell ......

...... Some memories burn themselves into the body, into the bones ...... and my body can also store peace and relaxation in every cell ......

...... My body can now make me even calmer ...... and my body can also store peace and relaxation in every cell ......

...... I now decide to never use violence again ......

## Emotional Orientation

...... I can now feel my own feelings better ...... and I let myself feel my painful emotions and process them completely inside ......

… … I also feel that I lacked self-confidence … … and I let myself feel my painful emotions and process them completely inside … …

… … I feel that I was bitter and frustrated … … and I let myself feel my painful emotions and process them completely inside … …

… … I feel old humiliations and degradations within me … … and I let myself feel my painful emotions and process them completely inside … …

… … I now decide to never use violence again … …

Behavioral Orientation

… … I am strong enough to act as I believe is right … … therefore I will leave situations of aggressive confrontation and avoid senseless violence from now on … …

… … I know that the use of violence was never right … … therefore I will leave situations of aggressive confrontation and avoid senseless violence from now on … …

… … I can control myself and pull myself together … … therefore I will leave situations of aggressive confrontation and avoid senseless violence from now on … …

… … I take full responsibility for my actions … … therefore I will leave situations of aggressive confrontation and avoid senseless violence from now on … …

… … I now decide to never use violence again … …

Reinforcement

… … I allow all suggestions to unfold their strongest effect now … … and therefore I truly end the time of violence and decide for a responsible and constructive life … …

… … As soon as I return to my everyday life, I can optimally benefit from this hypnosis and change everything … … and therefore I truly end the time of violence and decide for a responsible and constructive life … …

… … I say no to all forms of violence, and I clearly say yes to a peaceful, constructive life and coexistence with other people … … This is my path … … Yes, this is my path … …

# #7

## Contact and Relief

... ... You are not only a perpetrator ... ... You are also a victim ... ... You have dealt a lot with your actions and you know your responsibility ... ... and you have asked yourself what actually made you a perpetrator ... ... You yourself were once a victim of violence ... ... As a child, you were beaten, perhaps you also had to witness violence against others that you could not protect ... ... just as you could not protect yourself ... ... Maybe you tried, or maybe you did not dare ... ... You had no chance ... ... As a child, you wished it would stop ... ... Later, you became a perpetrator yourself ... ... adopting the system of violence ... ... You have been judged by many, perhaps also by courts ... ... and finally also by yourself ... ... Your childhood experiences did not force you to become a perpetrator ... ... but they contributed to making violence easier to apply, to lowering your threshold for using hard violence ... ... The good thing is that you can learn more from your past ... ... You can learn from your violent past how to do better ... ... better than the perpetrators in your life ... ... better than you did as a perpetrator ... ... You can learn to free yourself ... ...

## Self-Forgiveness and Comfort

... ... Back then, you were defenseless against the violence ... ... You needed someone to help you ... ... someone to protect you or get you out of there ... ... a savior in distress ... ... But there was no one ... ... It was a terrible time, and you were completely innocent as a child ... ... But children always end up blaming themselves ... ... You know that ... ... Over time, you thought it was your fault that you were beaten ... ... You may have thought you deserved it or were worth nothing more than to be beaten ... ... Today, you know that this is not true ... ... You were innocent ... ... Today, you can give yourself protection and comfort ... ... you can help yourself ... ... but you do not need violence against others for that, because other people are not your threat today ... ... The demons of the past are your threat ... ... the fear of weakness ... ... the fear of humiliation ... ... the fear of beatings and defeats ... ... Today, you can recognize these feelings again ... ... the feelings behind the violence ... ... maybe completely different feelings ... ... loneliness ... ... sadness ... ... helplessness ... ... or feelings that only you know and feel ... ... Accept these feelings and let them out ... ... Free yourself from them ... ... [approximately 20 seconds of silence] ... ...

Resolution and Self-Agreement

+++ Variant 1: General Use of Violence +++

... ... It is now time to look at and process your past ... ... It is time to engage with your old feelings ... ... with the repressed experiences and fears ... ... with all that you have never told anyone ... ... I know that you are afraid of it ... ... I know that you are afraid you would show weakness and be judged for your thoughts and feelings ... ... But now is the time to look at all that and take this risk ... ... If you honestly look into your innermost self, you know that you are the one who has this judgment ... ... You yourself think that you are worthless and that no one wants to see who you really are ... ... who you are behind the violence ... ... even though you would love to show it ... ... So, gather your courage and engage with it ... ... Show your true face ... ... Try to accept and understand yourself, because then the violence will be over forever ... ...

+++ End of Variant 1 +++

### +++ Variant 2: Convicted Violent Offenders +++

… … It is now time to look at and process your past … … It is time to engage with your old feelings … … to recognize that you find a way out of crimes by processing your past … … Yes, it is important to show respect to the victims and tell them that you are sorry and that you regret it … … You may have done this in one way or another … … But it is also important to confront yourself and your past, because only then can you truly end the violence … … I know that you are afraid of it … … I know that you are afraid you would show weakness and be judged for your thoughts and feelings … … But now is the time to look at all that and take this risk … … If you honestly look into your innermost self, you know that you are the one who has this judgment … … You yourself think that you are worthless and that no one wants to see who you really are … … and that is harder than any court judgment could be … … So, gather your courage and engage with it … … Show your true face … … Try to accept and understand yourself, because then the violence will be over forever … …

+++ End of Variant 2 +++

Success and Reinforcement

… … Well done … … Enough has been done for today … … You understand, I am sure of it … … You are now ready to take another, deeper step of self-encounter … … You are now ready to face your past … … And you know that you are not alone in this … … Allow yourself to enjoy the peace a little more now, because the healing peace of the trance helps you gather strength for your further journey … … for the path to your liberation … …

# #8

## Goal Formulation and Will Strengthening

... ... I engage with my own past and accept my history ... ... because I know that this is the only way to free myself from the power of the past ... ...

... ... I engage with my own past and accept my history ... ... because I want to finally process the past events and be free again ... ...

... ... I engage with my own past and accept my history ... ... because this is how I can be free in the present and never need violence again ... ...

... ... I engage with my own past and accept my history ... ... because I finally want to put an end to the violence ... ...

## Thought Orientation

### +++ Variant 1: General Use of Violence +++

… … I know that I can and must process the past internally … … and therefore I also let go of aggression internally and remain outwardly calm … …

… … I know that I can and must process the past internally … … and therefore I can also meet the people around me peacefully and calmly … …

… … I know that I can and must process the past internally … … and therefore I can also better ignore external provocations … …

… … I know that I can and must process the past internally … … and therefore I do exactly that and dissolve the violence within me … …

… … I accept my life and make something good out of it … …

+++ End of Variant 1 +++

### +++ Variant 2: Convicted Violent Offenders +++

... ... I know that I must face my demons of violence ... ... and therefore I immediately and forever stop being a demon for others ... ...

... ... I know that I must face my demons of violence ... ... and therefore I also take my conviction as a chance for a new beginning ... ...

... ... I know that I must face my demons of violence ... ... and therefore I can also better ignore external provocations ... ...

... ... I know that I must face my demons of violence ... ... and therefore I do exactly that and stop the senseless violence against people ... ...

... ... I accept my life and make something good out of it ... ...

+++ End of Variant 2 +++

## Somatic Orientation

... ... I take advantage of the benefits of physical relaxation at this moment ... ... and consciously feel how pleasant this peace and relaxation are ... ...

... ... I take advantage of the benefits of physical relaxation at this moment ... ... and imagine how liberating it will be when this peace becomes my basic feeling ... ...

... ... I take advantage of the benefits of physical relaxation at this moment ... ... and imagine situations where I lost control and remain calm now ... ...

... ... I take advantage of the benefits of physical relaxation at this moment ... ... and I think of humiliations and pain that I have suffered myself, and remain calm ... ...

... ... I accept my life and make something good out of it ... ...

## Emotional Orientation

... ... I feel the pain and hatred of the past and accept these feelings as my own ... ... and with that, they become lighter and gradually dissolve ... ...

... ... I feel the pain and hatred of the past and accept them as my feelings ... ... and with that, it is completely clear that I no longer direct them against others ... ...

... ... I feel the pain and hatred of the past and accept these feelings as my own ... ... and with that, I feel the sadness and loneliness behind the pain ... ...

... ... I feel the pain and hatred of the past and accept these feelings as my own ... ... and with that, I truly tear down the wall of violence ... ...

... ... I accept my life and make something good out of it ... ...


Behavioral Orientation

... ... I accept life and my personal history ... ... because the people I have harmed with violence are not to blame ... ...

... ... I accept life and my personal history ... ... because only in this way can I make something good out of my own experience ... ...

...... I accept life and my personal history ...... because only in this way can I make inner peace and the violence will end forever ......

...... I accept life and my personal history ...... because I have no other story – I make the best out of it ......

...... I accept my life and make something good out of it ......

Reinforcement

...... I now reclaim my life step by step, my non-violent and constructive life ...... and with that also my self-confidence and my dignity ......

...... I now reclaim my life step by step, my non-violent and constructive life ...... and with that, I also give the people around me a better and more peaceful life ......

...... I now reclaim my life step by step, my non-violent and constructive life ...... because I end the violence today and every day ...... I truly end the violence forever ...... Never again violence ...... Never again violence ......

# #9

## Goal Formulation and Will Strengthening

... ... I dive deep into the trance and thus deep into my innermost self ... ... because this is the only way I can finally recognize and process my deep feelings ... ...

... ... I accept all suggestions of this hypnosis constructively ... ... because this is the only way I can finally recognize and process my deep feelings ... ...

... ... I am ready to look deep into my innermost self ... ... because this is the only way I can finally recognize and process my deep feelings ... ...

... ... Today, I look deeper into my emotions than ever before ... ... because this is the only way I can finally recognize and process my deep feelings ... ...

## Thought Orientation

### +++ Variant 1: General Use of Violence +++

... ... I remember violence in my childhood ... ... and precisely because of this, I want to make no one else a victim ... ...

... ... I myself was a victim of violence in my childhood ... ... and precisely because of this, I want to make no one else a victim ... ...

... ... I know that my victims had nothing to do with my history of violence ... ... and precisely because of this, I want to make no one else a victim ... ...

... ... I know that there have already been too many victims ... ... and precisely because of this, I want to make no one else a victim ... ...

... ... I accept my history and consciously hand it over to the past ... ...

+++ End of Variant 1 +++

### +++ Variant 2: Convicted Violent Offenders +++

... ... I remember violence in my childhood ... ... and precisely because of this, I realize that I never had the right to direct violence against others in the present ... ...

... ... I myself was a victim of violence in my childhood ... ... and precisely because of this, I realize that I never had the right to direct violence against others in the present ... ...

... ... My victims have nothing to do with my history ... ... and precisely because of this, I realize that I never had the right to direct violence against others in the present ... ...

... ... I know that there have already been too many victims ... ... and precisely because of this, I realize that I never had the right to direct violence against others in the present ... ...

... ... I accept my history and consciously hand it over to the past ... ...

+++ End of Variant 2 +++

## Somatic Orientation

… … My body is now completely calm, and this calm spreads further … … and in this calm, I can finally process the past … …

… … With every breath, my calm goes even deeper … … and in this calm, I can finally process the past … …

… … More and more, this calm becomes my actual basic feeling … … and in this calm, I can finally process the past … …

… … More and more, I find memories of violence in this calm … … and in this calm, I can finally process the past … …

… … I accept my history and consciously hand it over to the past … …


## Emotional Orientation

… … I can now feel my own feelings better … … and I accept all repressed feelings again and process them inside … …

... ... I also feel that there are still many once repressed feelings rising now ... ... and I accept all repressed feelings again and process them inside ... ...

... ... I feel that all memories are associated with intense feelings ... ... and I accept all repressed feelings again and process them inside ... ...

... ... I feel fear and disappointment deep inside me ... ... and I accept all repressed feelings again and process them inside ... ...

... ... I accept my history and consciously hand it over to the past ... ...

### Behavioral Orientation

... ... I know that violence belongs to my past and only to the past ... ... therefore I bring all memories now to the place of experience and become free ...

... ... I know that violence was never right, not even the violence against me ... ... therefore I bring all memories now to the place of experience and become free ... ...

... ... I know that I can shape the present myself ... ... therefore I bring all memories now to the place of experience and become free ... ...

... ... I take full responsibility for my actions ... ... therefore I bring all memories now to the place of experience and become free ... ...

... ... I accept my history and consciously hand it over to the past ... ...

Reinforcement

... ... I know that I cannot erase my history, but it does not define me ... ... and therefore I accept the painful memories as my experiences and make the best out of it ... ... a life without violence ... ...

... ... I know that here and today and every day I can consciously shape my life without violence ... ... and therefore I accept the painful memories as my experiences and make the best out of it ... ... a life without violence ... ...

... ... I say no to all forms of violence, and I clearly say yes to a peaceful, constructive life and coexistence with other people ... ... This is my path ... ... Yes, this is my path ... ...

# #10

### Arriving in the Land of Dreams

... ... Today you will embark on a very special journey ... ... a journey to a place you have never seen before, yet you have been there many times ... ... in the land of your dreams ... ... Feel the rhythm of your body moving up and down with your breath like a wave ... ... Imagine the waves of your body carrying you away, just like the waves of the ocean could ... ... You go to the land of dreams ... ... In this land, you become an explorer who can find everything ... ... because everything has always been there and can be seen when the right time comes ... ... You set off ... ...

### Confrontation, Clarification, and Creative Reorientation

... ... You discover a high iron fence that runs through the dreamland ... ... On your side of the fence, everything is green and alive ... ... You stand on a lush meadow, there are trees with ripe fruits, flowers, and bushes, and friendly animals ... ... You hear birds chirping and can enjoy the beauty of life and nature on your side ... ... You go to the fence ... ... On the other side of the fence, everything is barren and desolate, and a huge gray shadow lies over the land behind the fence ... ... The stormy wind on the other side blows gray sand and dust across the land, but on your side, everything is peaceful and beautiful ... ... The fence runs like a border through the land of dreams ... ... a border that separates two worlds ... ... And through the gray sandstorm, a figure approaches, wearing a dark heavy coat and a hood pulled over the head ... ... The figure steps up to the fence ... ... You recognize the perpetrator of your childhood ... ... the person you once loved, who brought violence into your life, and without your wanting it, became your role model ... ... Motionless, they remain on their side of the fence ... ... Here in the land of dreams, only you decide what is possible ... ... No one you do not invite can cross the fence and be with you in the land of dreams ... ... not even them ... ... This person is not here for their own sake ... ... It does not matter what their motives were or what their story was ... ... Like you, they also have a land of their dreams, as we all do, where they can find their story if they are ready for it ... ... Here it is only about you and your violent acts ... ... You think about what you want to say to them ... ... Just tell them about the feelings and the fear you once had ... ... back when violence was still a daily occurrence ... ... Also tell them the feelings that perhaps only you know, that you have never talked to anyone about, but that you might now feel as a memory ... ... Take your time to tell this person about it ... ... If you want, tell them about it, if you want, scream it at them ... ... Do it as your feelings dictate, because now you do not have to fulfill anything, keep your composure ... ... You are not here to forgive, but to free yourself ... ... Say now in the land of dreams what you want or need to say ... ... I am with you and will give you some time ... ... [Now make a perceived one-minute pause and let the client go into inner contact to feel and internally express their feelings.] ... ...

... ... You still stand at the fence between the worlds, and the person on the other side turns into a stone sculpture ... ... They can no longer move, can do nothing to you, can do nothing at all because the time from back then is long gone ... ... ... ... The world on the other side of the fence is a shadow of the past ... ... Whatever the perpetrator of back then could do today, if they are still alive, the past cannot be changed ... ... just as you cannot undo your violent acts ...

... They are part of your history ... ... The part of this person on the shadow side, whom you once loved and perhaps still love because they were without violence and horror ... ... this part lives somewhere in the land of your dreams, as color, as sound, or as an image of nature ... ... But the part of violence that scared you, that made you a perpetrator yourself, stands as a stone sculpture beyond the fence and crumbles before your eyes into dust that is blown away by the wind ... ...

Mindfulness and Self-Loyalty

+++ Variant 1: General Use of Violence +++

... ... Then you sink to the ground and let the uncried tears of the past come up ... ... You now allow all feelings and let them out ... ... the pain ... ... the fear ... ... the insults ... ... the loneliness ... ... the longing for love ... ... or the feeling that you now feel the most, whatever it is ... ... You cry in the land of dreams ... ... until the last tear is shed ... ... [approximately 20 seconds of silence] ... ... You let go of all the old inner pains with your tears ... ... and you let go of the violence because you realize that it was just a wall in front of your own pains ... ... You realize that you never wanted to feel so small and weak again and that is why you often used violence ... ... Somehow what the perpetrator of your childhood once did became a little more bearable ... ... a little less horrible ... ... But it was horrible, and what you did was horrible for your victims ... ... With your tears, you end this vicious cycle ... ... Today, you do what the perpetrator of your childhood never managed to do ... ... You end the violence ... ... because you are strong enough to achieve that ... ...

+++ End of Variant 1 +++

+++ Variant 2: Convicted Violent Offenders +++

... ... Then you think of the violence you yourself have used ... ... You think of the crimes you have committed ... ... You think of your victims and sink to the ground and let the uncried tears of the past come up ... ... You now allow all feelings and let them out ... ... the pain ... ... the fear ... ... the insults ... ... the loneliness ... ... the longing for love ... ... or the feeling that you now feel the most, whatever it is ... ... You cry in the land of dreams ... ... until the last tear is shed ... ... [approximately 20 seconds of silence] ... ... You let go of all the old inner pains with your tears ... ... and you let go of the violence because you realize that it was just a wall in front of your own pains ... ... You realize that you never wanted to feel so small and weak again and that is why you became so violent that you even ended up in court and were convicted for it ... [preferably something specific ... spent half a year in prison / received a suspended sentence etc. ...] ... You regret what you did, but you cannot change it anymore ... ... But you can do something very important ... ... You can end the violence ... ... With your tears, you end the vicious cycle of violence ... ... Today, you do what the perpetrator of your childhood never managed to do ... ... You end the violence ... ... because you are strong enough to achieve that ... ...

+++ End of Variant 2 +++

... ... Then you stand up and continue walking ... ... Step by step, you go towards the horizon because that is where your future begins, your non-violent future ... ... and the future begins in the next moment ... ... with the next breath ... ... You are in the land of dreams and thus in your own feeling ... ... because the land of dreams is deep within you ... ... It has always been there ... ... I am just telling you about it ... ...

Distribution, publication, and copying in any form are prohibited and subject to damages.

Copying, publishing, and sharing with third parties are only permitted with the written consent of the author. Please observe the notes on copyright and usage.

Distribution, publication, and copying in any form are prohibited and subject to damages.

## Overview of All Titles in the Series "Ten Hypnoses"

Volume 1: Smoking Cessation
Volume 2: Anxiety and Restlessness
Volume 3: Burnout
Volume 4: Reducing Overweight
Volume 5: Coping with the Past
Volume 6: Suicidal Thoughts and Attempts
Volume 7: Psycho-Oncology
Volume 8: Obsessions and Tics
Volume 9: Self-Confidence and Decision-Making
Volume 10: Grief Work
Volume 11: Psychosomatics
Volume 12: Chronic Pain
Volume 13: Depressive Thoughts
Volume 14: Panic Attacks
Volume 15: Domestic Violence, Victim Support
Volume 16: Post-Traumatic Stress
Volume 17: Exam Anxiety and Stage Fright
Volume 18: Anti-Violence Training, Offender Support
Volume 19: Addiction Tendencies
Volume 20: Social Phobia and Fear of Contact
Volume 21: Nail Biting
Volume 22: Self-Awareness and Self-Love
Volume 23: Teeth Grinding and Night Clenching
Volume 24: Feelings of Guilt
Volume 25: Fear in Crowds
Volume 26: Fear of Flying, Aviophobia
Volume 27: Fear in Enclosed Spaces, Claustrophobia
Volume 28: Tinnitus, Ear Noises
Volume 29: Fear of Heights
Volume 30: Neurodermatitis

Copying, publishing, and sharing with third parties are only permitted with the written consent of the author. Please observe the notes on copyright and usage.

Volume 31: Finding Inner Balance
Volume 32: Overcoming Loneliness
Volume 33: Fear of Illness, Hypochondria
Volume 34: Anticipatory Anxiety, Fear of Fear
Volume 35: Jealousy in Relationships
Volume 36: Driving Anxiety
Volume 37: New Start after Separation
Volume 38: Fear of Injections
Volume 39: Heart Anxiety Neurosis
Volume 40: Overcoming Resentment and Anger
Volume 41: Resolving Blockages and Positive Thinking
Volume 42: Stress Reduction, Stress Management
Volume 43: Body Relaxation
Volume 44: Deep Relaxation
Volume 45: Fear of the Dark
Volume 46: Falling Asleep and Staying Asleep
Volume 47: Compulsive Buying
Volume 48: Restless Legs Syndrome
Volume 49: Bulimia
Volume 50: Anorexia
Volume 51: Overcoming Nightmares
Volume 52: Imagined Deformity
Volume 53: Overcoming Distrust, Finding Trust
Volume 54: Processing Failures
Volume 55: Humiliation, Emotional Hurt
Volume 56: Distressing Compassion, Vicarious Suffering
Volume 57: Self-Forgiveness
Volume 58: Self-Awareness, Self-Confidence
Volume 59: Saying No
Volume 60: Assertiveness
Volume 61: Setting Boundaries and Self-Assertion
Volume 62: Decision-Making Ability

Volume 63: Success Orientation
Volume 64: Ruminating, Circular Thinking
Volume 65: Accepting Pregnancy
Volume 66: Birth Preparation
Volume 67: Spiritual Opening
Volume 68: Joy of Life and Inner Lightness
Volume 69: Patience and Inner Peace
Volume 70: Fibromyalgia and Rheumatism
Volume 71: Irritable Bowel Syndrome, Crohn's Disease
Volume 72: Fear of Nausea, Emetophobia
Volume 73: Stuttering and Cluttering, Speech Flow Disorders
Volume 74: Concentration and Knowledge Anchoring
Volume 75: Vitality and Spontaneity
Volume 76: Searching for Meaning and Finding Goals
Volume 77: Life Crises, Life Events
Volume 78: Workaholism, Goal Obsession
Volume 79: Helper Syndrome, Helpless Helpers
Volume 80: Medication Abuse
Volume 81: Gambling Addiction
Volume 82: Internet Addiction, Smartphone Addiction
Volume 83: Hoarding Disorder, Compulsive Collecting
Volume 84: Conspiracy Thoughts, Overvalued Ideas
Volume 85: Fear of Operations and Treatments
Volume 86: Fear of Aging
Volume 87: Travel Anxiety
Volume 88: Anxiety When Urinating, Paruresis
Volume 89: Fear of Intimacy and Togetherness
Volume 90: Fear of Blushing
Volume 91: Coming Out in Homosexuality
Volume 92: Charisma Training
Volume 93: Migraines and Chronic Headaches
Volume 94: Overcoming Allergies, Bronchial Asthma

Volume 95: Normalizing Blood Pressure
Volume 96: Compulsive Perfectionism
Volume 97: Sports Hypnosis, Motivation
Volume 98: Sports Hypnosis, Performance Enhancement
Volume 99: Determination and Focus
Volume 100: Encountering the Inner Child
Volume 101: Cravings, Binge Eating
Volume 102: Stimulating Metabolism
Volume 103: Bipolar Mood Swings
Volume 104: Borderline, Identity Crises
Volume 105: Hypomania, Euphoria, Mania
Volume 106: Restlessness, Agitation
Volume 107: Nervous Breakdown
Volume 108: Adjustment Disorders
Volume 109: Self-Alienation, Depersonalization
Volume 110: Ending Self-Pity
Volume 111: Primary Gain of Illness
Volume 112: Secondary Gain of Illness
Volume 113: Bullying, Victim Support
Volume 114: Letting Go of Envy and Jealousy
Volume 115: Fear of Spiders, Arachnophobia
Volume 116: Fear of Dogs or Cats
Volume 117: Fear of Strangers, Xenophobia
Volume 118: Excessive Worries, Generalized Anxiety
Volume 119: Strengthening Sense of Responsibility
Volume 120: Unrequited Love, Heartache
Volume 121: Work-Life Balance
Volume 122: Letting Go of Unattainable Goals
Volume 123: Allowing and Accepting Help
Volume 124: Letting Go of Adult Children
Volume 125: Tourette Syndrome
Volume 126: Life Changes and New Starts

Volume 127: Accepting Life in a Wheelchair
Volume 128: Understanding and Overcoming Homesickness
Volume 129: Understanding and Overcoming Wanderlust
Volume 130: Dizziness, Meniere's Disease
Volume 131: Overcoming Aggression
Volume 132: Cutting and Self-Harm
Volume 133: Hair Pulling, Trichotillomania
Volume 134: Postpartum Depression
Volume 135: For Relatives of Dementia Patients
Volume 136: Self-Harm, Artificial Disorders
Volume 137: Activating Self-Healing Powers
Volume 138: Preventing Depression Relapse
Volume 139: Reactive Psychoses, Follow-Up
Volume 140: Obsessive Thoughts and Impulses
Volume 141: Compulsive Checking
Volume 142: Compulsive Counting, Symmetry Obsession
Volume 143: Compulsive Washing, Cleanliness Obsession
Volume 144: Compulsive Questioning
Volume 145: Dissociative Paralysis
Volume 146: Phantom Pain
Volume 147: Overcoming Complaining
Volume 148: Hay Fever, Pollen Allergy
Volume 149: Sexual Abuse, Victim Support
Volume 150: Standing Strong Against Sexism, #metoo
Volume 151: Binge Eating
Volume 152: Overcoming Thoughts of Revenge
Volume 153: Detachment from the Aggressor, Stockholm Syndrome
Volume 154: Courage to Separate
Volume 155: Chronic Fatigue, Exhaustion
Volume 156: Fear of the Future, Existential Anxiety
Volume 157: Excessive Worry About Children
Volume 158: Fear of Failure

Volume 159: Ending Distrust and Control
Volume 160: Dejection, Dysphoria
Volume 161: Boreout, Chronic Boredom
Volume 162: Bipolar Disorders, Relapse Prevention
Volume 163: Mania, Relapse Prevention
Volume 164: Nihilism, Feelings of Worthlessness
Volume 165: Thumb Sucking
Volume 166: Being Brave
Volume 167: Being Proud
Volume 168: Overcoming Shyness
Volume 169: Being Able to Delegate Responsibility
Volume 170: Being Able to Show Emotions
Volume 171: Letting Go of Guilt, Victim Support
Volume 172: Processing Guilt, Offender Support
Volume 173: Mood Swings, Cyclothymia
Volume 174: Lack of Drive, Vital Sadness
Volume 175: Hearing Voices with Reality Reference
Volume 176: Confident Communication
Volume 177: Standing Up for Oneself
Volume 178: Taking New Paths
Volume 179: Confident Job Application
Volume 180: No Longer Being Taken Advantage Of
Volume 181: End of Submissiveness
Volume 182: Depressive Numbness
Volume 183: Mood Drops, Affective Incontinence
Volume 184: Mood Instability
Volume 185: Somatoform Disorders
Volume 186: Stomach Ulcer, Psychosomatic
Volume 187: Accepting Amputation
Volume 188: Overcoming and Letting Go of Hatred
Volume 189: Ending Accusations
Volume 190: Allowing Tears, Being Able to Cry

Volume 191: Finding and Sorting Repressed Feelings
Volume 192: Somatoform Pain
Volume 193: Living Autonomously
Volume 194: Anhedonia, Joylessness
Volume 195: Persistent Sadness
Volume 196: Obesity, Food Addiction
Volume 197: Parents of Abused Children
Volume 198: Letting Go and Letting Be
Volume 199: Childhood Sexual Abuse
Volume 200: Fear of Loss

www.ingramcontent.com/pod-product-compliance
Lightning Source LLC
Chambersburg PA
CBHW030452220526
45464CB00006B/2505